Elucidating
SEXUALLY TRANSMITTED INFECTIONS
2nd Edition

(Epidemiology, Aetiology, Diagnosis, Management, and Prevention)

Dorcas Obiri-Yeboah
(MB.ChB, PhD)

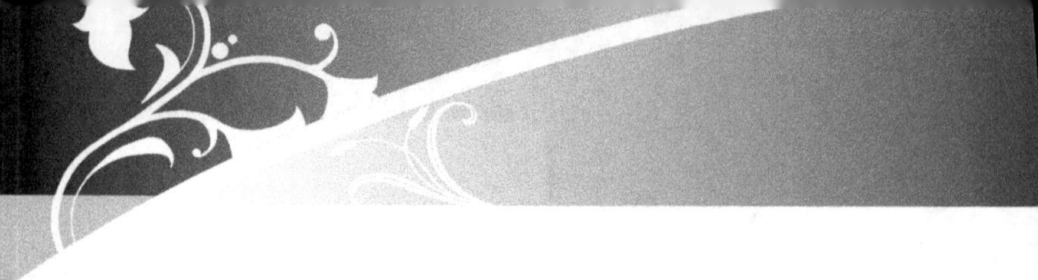

Typeset in Helvetica Neue and ITC Berkeley Oldstyle

Icon Publishing Ltd
P. O. Box OD 972
Odorkor, Accra
Ghana

ISBN: 978-9988-53-454-7

Other Books by the Author

Medical Microbiology Simplified
(ISBN: 9789988856779)

Medical Microbiology Simplified
(2nd Edition)
(ISBN: 9789988148652)

Elucidating Sexually Transmitted Infections
(ISBN: 9789988856724)

In Treasured Honour of

My daughter, Castella Obiri-Yeboah

Contents

Foreword

This book is the result of years of academic study, teaching and research on the complex subject of sexually transmitted infections (STIs). With the discovery of syphilis in ancient Egyptian mummies, sexually transmitted diseases are probably as nearly as old as history could account for the existence of the human race. The fact that sex is the medium of transmission of these infections makes it a difficult to discuss subject in many cultures where discussions on sexuality and sexual activity are sacrosanct. The social construct and interpretation of societal norms relating to sex and infections relating to the sexual act, makes it difficult to deal with even amongst the most educated. The advent of newer STIs like the Human Immunodeficiency Virus (HIV) renewed the fueling of stigma and discrimination which make disclosure difficult and negatively affect the health-seeking behavior of persons who may be infected with or exposed to any STIs.

Sexually transmitted infections are of global significance with an estimated daily infection rate of nearly one million globally. A high percentage of these infections are never detected, remain asymptomatic, unreported, undertreated, mismanaged or go untreated. Thus STIs ultimately will yield their undesired result of complications which could result in life-long debilitation for adults, children, the newborn and even the unborn. To the extent that sex is directly linked to human reproduction, STIs may negatively affect the reproductive life of individuals and couples, often with the associated complexity of socio-religious connotations. Issues of breakdown in marriages, infertility and mistrust often complicate the purely biological issue caused by these microscopic organisms that find the expression of transmissibility through a mostly pleasurable natural human activity as sex. This book draws deep, and looks much closer, searches intently but above all throw light on the subject of STIs in a structures layer-by-layer approach that should make it easier for students, teachers and healthcare practitioners to make the most use of without any lurking doubts as to clarity.

Interestingly the title of this well researched and excellently written book, "Elucidating Sexually Transmitted Infections' succinctly tells the nature of the subject-matter it sought to address. For if there is any infection such as is common to mankind that has been hidden and survived generations in all countries of the world, that is mostly acquired through a most natural human interaction, that is linked to the act of perpetuation of the human race, that is acquired mostly under cover of darkness, that is most likely not to be disclosed, that would most probably go untreated on account of its asymptomatic tendency, that could have dire consequences of complications, that has serious social and religious ramifications, then it should be none other than sexually transmitted infections.

Prevention and public health interventions take centre-stage in this book and personally, that gladdens my heart, as we cannot be unconcerned about the almost one million daily new infections occurring globally just because we can identify causative organisms, understand the epidemiology, make diagnosis and effectively manage those already infected. Focusing the beam on interventions aimed at reducing new infections and minimizing complications of the infected is commendable. The structured approach adopted in this book makes it easy to follow, as it offers students as well as teachers and healthcare practitioners a concise guide to the diagnoses, management and prevention of sexually transmitted infections.

The author surely has done an excellent work which is a reflection of the amalgamation of her passion, resilience, hard work and quest for treading new grounds through research.

Dr. Bernard Dornoo
June, 2018

Links to online profile of the author:
- *https://scholar.google.com/citations?user=cgs34h-UAAAAJ&hl=en*
- *https://www.researchgate.net/profile/Dorcas_Obiri-Yeboah*
- *http://uccsms.edu.gh/obiriyeboah/*

Acknowledgements

I am profoundly grateful to my mentors, Prof. Harold Amonoo-Kuofi (Founding Dean of The School of Medical Sciences, University of Cape Coast), Prof. Yaw Adu-Sarkodie, the late Prof. E. H. Frimpong, (both of the Department of Clinical Microbiology, School of Medical Sciences, Kwame Nkrumah University of Science and Technology, Ghana), Prof. Philippe Mayaud (Department of Clinical Research, London School of Hygiene and Tropical Medicine, United Kingdom), and Prof. Jacques Simpore (University of Ouagadougou, Director of CERBA/LABIOGENE and Rector of Saint Thomas d'Aquin University, Burkina Faso) who have contributed in various ways to my academic and professional development. Your support and encouragement which in no small way contributed to the realization of this dream is truly appreciated.

My sincere appreciation goes to all the various members of staff of the School of Medical Sciences, University of Cape Coast who have been very supportive and played diverse roles in contributing to ensure this book was completed.

A special thanks to Dr. Bernard Dornoo (Medical Director, University Health Services, University of Professional Studies, Accra, Ghana and former Head of Clinical Care Unit, National HIV/AIDS/ STIs Control Program, Ghana) for the great work done in reviewing this book. Your contribution is very much appreciated. You had the hardest task. This book would not have been complete without your inputs. The final product is a result of your good work done. Thank you.

Introduction to the Second Edition

This second edition has been necessitated by a number of factors. The most important factor has been the need for this book to be up to date keeping in mind revision of guidelines and recommendations from relevant health agencies particularly the World Health Organization (WHO). Thus, some chapters have seen major changes, for example, the Chapter 11 on the Human immunodeficiency Virus (HIV) has undergone significant revision particularly in the area of the diagnosis and antiretroviral therapy protocols backed by strong scientific evidence. Chapter 4 and 6 on Gonorrhoea and syphilis respectively has additional details and recommendations on the treatment guidelines. Some chapters have also been improved by making the points clearer and providing some additional information (e.g. Chapters 3 and 9). There has also been some formatting to improve the flow of thought for some chapters. It is hope that all these revisions have made this edition better.

Introduction to Sexually Transmitted Infections

It is estimated that there are over 370 million new cases of 1 of these 4 (gonorrhoea, syphilis, chlamydia and trichomoniasis) sexually transmitted infections (STIs) worldwide every year. More than 70% of such cases are said to occur in developing countries with the consequent economic burden. Over the centuries, STIs have remained of health importance but this interest increased tremendously in recent times due to the emergence of the Human Immunodeficiency Virus (HIV). Efforts to control the spread of HIV brought to the fore the importance of all STIs associated potential to increase the risk of acquisition and progression of HIV. Thus controlling other STIs also controls the spread of HIV and hence its impact. STIs are also important because of the link between such infections and adverse maternal and birth outcomes including stillbirths, neonatal deaths and others. Syphilis in particular has contributed significantly to these. Thus any effort aimed at improving maternal and birth outcomes, must of necessity include enhancement of STI services.

Why the high STI burden?

This question is simply answered with one word; SEX! Sexual and reproductive activities are necessary for the preservation of all species including humans and will thus continue to be part of the human existence. And to the extent that sexual and reproductive organs are closely knit, the risk of acquisition of STIs would continue to transcend the human race from the cradle to the grave. This instinctive, pleasurable, reproductive human behaviour is therefore, practically very difficult to regulate both intrinsically and extrinsically.

Beyond the context of instinct, pleasure and reproduction, sex has within certain parameters continued to be viewed, offered or procured as a 'commodity' which is utilized or engaged in for various reasons, acceptable or unacceptable, moral or immoral, legal or illegal. Many socio-cultural factors and behavioural inclinations may lead to people engaging in sexual activities with more than 1 person in their life time or even within a shorter time-frame. It is well known how economic factors and desire for economic gain has for centuries been a driving force for the engagement of sex for financial gain (e.g. Commercial sex work) and other favours or exploitation (e.g. In the workplace). The factors that mainly fuel these, include economic status, gender inequalities and cultural norms in mainly developing countries (e.g. polygamy, widowhood rights etc.). Worse of all, sex is sometimes forcefully and illegally 'demanded and taken' from particularly but not limited to females in cases of rape and defilement, which even put survivors of such abuse at greater risk of acquiring STIs. The sexual activities and act themselves have evolved over the centuries with practices which were previously frown upon in generations past now becoming common with all the associated risks in this generation. Currently aside peno-vaginal sex, other forms of sexual acts (oral and anal sex) are becoming common and with the associated increasing risk of STI acquisition by several folds when practices without additional protective practices.

In addition to these social and behavioural factors, the STI burden also remains high because re-infection associated with most recorded STIs cases. There is lack or inadequate acquired immunity for most STIs hence people can get re-infected by the same, most often, asymptomatic sexual partner or by another sexual partner.

Types of STIs

Various microorganisms (over 30 bacteria, parasites and viruses) are said to be transmissible through semen, oral and vaginal secretions from an infected person to the sexual partner. The efficiency of transmission is affected by many factors including the type of sexual act, the particular microorganism involved, and host factors. About 8 of these (in bold) have the highest incidence globally and hence requires the greatest attention. These microorganisms include:

1. Bacteria: ***Neisseria gonorrhoeae*** (gonorrhoea), ***Chlamydia trachomatis***, ***Treponema pallidum*** (syphilis), *Haemophilus ducreyi* (chancroid), *Klebsiella granulomatis* (donovanosis).

2. Viruses: ***Herpes simplex virus (type1 and 2), hepatitis B virus, human papillomavirus,*** *Molluscum contagiosum*, ***HIV (type1 and 2).***

3. Fungus: *Candida species*

4. Protozoa: ***Trichomonas vaginalis*** *(trichomoniasis), Giardia lamblia, Entamoeba histolytica,*

5. Ecto-parasites: *Pthirus pubis* (pubic lice), *Sarcoptes scabiei* (scabies)

Impact of STIs

Generally STIs are recognized to have negative impact on the individuals, their families, communities, and countries. STIs are associated with high mortality and morbidity and may have varied impact including the following:

- Impact on reproductive health: many STIs (Chlamydia infection and gonorrhoea particularly) increase the risk of pelvic inflammatory diseases, ectopic pregnancies, infertility, spontaneous abortions, and preterm deliveries. Females are disproportionately the worse affected for many reasons which include biological and socio-cultural factors.

- Impact on neonatal and child health: neonatal infections lead to complications for the developing foetus and neonates. The associated mortality and morbidity is high particularly in developing countries. Most surviving children have to live with complications like mental retardation, blindness and deafness.

- Facilitation of HIV transmission and acquisition thus resulting in high HIV prevalence in countries with high STI burden as seen in Africa. Syphilis and herpes are of particular interest.

- Facilitation of progression of HIV infection to AIDS: it is established that viral replication increases in the presence of other STIs and this result in rapid clinical progression

- HIV also increases the persistence and progression of other STIs such as human papillomavirus (HPV) and herpes simplex virus (HSV).

- Development of cancers with associated mortality, morbidity and economic impact: HPV associated cervical and oropharyngeal cancer, HIV associated Kaposi's sarcoma etc.

2

Approaches to the Diagnosis and Management of Sexually Transmitted Infections

Prompt diagnosis of STIs is essential to enable effective management of cases. While there are different approaches developed for the diagnosis of STIs, a detailed clinical history and thorough physical examination is essential in all cases. Since this encounter with patients will require them to talk about sensitive matters, it is essential that clinicians provide conducive environment for such consultations. A detailed history would not only reveal more about the current complaint but very importantly reveal details about risk factors which must be addressed. This will allow for a comprehensive case diagnosis and management. The main aims of management are:

1. To prevent or stop the transmission of STIs to other sexual partners
2. To prevent the development of complications in infected patients by curing them.
3. To reduce the risk of HIV transmission and acquisition
4. Prevent re-infection

To achieve these, various approaches have been proposed for STI diagnosis. These have been designed to ensure that STI diagnosis is possible in both resource-available and resource-constrained settings. The approaches to STI diagnosis are:

- Aetiologic approach
- Clinical approach
- Syndromic approach

Etiologic Approach to STI diagnosis

This approach is described as the "gold standard" as it is based on laboratory identification of the particular pathogen responsible for an STI. The World Health Organization (WHO) recommends that if possible this approach should be used except where there are laboratory and other challenges making it not feasible. The major advantages of this method are the fact that the most appropriate treatment can be offered to the confirmed patient and has the ability to identify asymptomatic but infected patients and manage them. However, the disadvantages include:

- Additional laboratory cost
- The need for a well resourced laboratory
- The need for personnel with the necessary knowledge and skills to perform the laboratory tests
- The high risk of loss to follow up as patients will have to return to the hospital on another day to get the results before treatment could be initiated.

Clinical Approach to STI diagnosis

This approach involves arriving at the diagnosis of a particular STI and treating it with the specific antibiotic based on the clinical presentation (history) and physical examination findings. The advantage it offers is the possibility to arrive at a diagnosis and offer treatment on the same day. There is however a high risk of over diagnosis and missed diagnosis as the experience of the clinician is the main diagnostic tool. In addition, asymptomatic patients will not be diagnosed by this approach.

Syndromic Approach to STI diagnosis

The WHO in an effort to address the limitations of the clinical and aetiologic approach to STI diagnosis developed and has advocated for the use of the syndromic approach especially at the lower levels of health delivery points. This method allows for the diagnosis of STIs based on symptoms (using flow charts) and groups them into syndromes for which treatment is then offered. For each syndrome, combinations of antibiotics are given for the possible organisms responsible for the symptoms (Table 2.1).

Advantages

- Allows for patients to be treated on the same clinic day.
- Sensitivity is high among symptomatic patients.
- Does not miss cases of mixed infections.
- It takes away the cost of laboratory investigations.
- The use of flow charts ensures that this can be implemented at very basic level of health care.

No.	STI SYNDROMES	ORGANISMS TREATED FOR
1.	Vaginal Discharge Syndrome	• *Neisseria gonorrhoeae* • *Chlamydia trachomatis* • *Trichomonas vaginalis* • *Candida albicans* • Bacterial vaginosis *(BV)*
2.	Urethral Discharge Syndrome	• *Neisseria gonorrhoeae* • *Chlamydia trachomatis* • *Trichomonas vaginalis* • *Mycoplasma genitalium*
3.	Genital Ulcer	• *Herpes simplex virus* • *Haemophilus ducreyi* • *Treponema pallidum* • *Calymmatobacterium granulomatis*
4.	Genital warts	• *Human papillomavirus* (commonly types 6 and 11)
5.	Scrotal Swelling	• *Neisseria gonorrhoeae* • *Chlamydia trachomatis* • *Mycoplasma genitalium*
6.	Lower Abdominal Pain (PID)	• *Neisseria gonorrhoeae* • *Chlamydia trachomatis*
7.	Neonatal Conjunctivitis	• *Neisseria gonorrhoeae* • *Chlamydia trachomatis*
8.	Inguinal Bubo	• *Chlamydia trachomatis,* L1,2, 3 • *Haemophilus ducreyi*
9.	Ano-rectal Related Syndromes	• *Neisseria gonorrhoeae* • *Chlamydia trachomatis* • *Herpes simplex virus* • *Treponema pallidum* • *Haemophilus ducreyi*

Table 2.1: STIs syndromes and associated causative organisms

Disadvantages

- There is an increased risk of over diagnosis of STIs.
- This approach will miss asymptomatic STI cases.
- The practice of using many antimicrobial agents has implications for:
  - High cost to patient,
  - Changes occurring in the vaginal microbial flora,
  - Potential increased drug side effects, and
  - Potential for development of drug resistance.

Targeted interventions

These interventions target people with recognized increased risk of STIs based on having multiple sexual partners or higher rates of sexual activity ("core groups"). Such groups include sex workers (CSWs) and men who have sex with men (MSMs). Sexual partners of these core groups are described as "bridging population" because they are a link between these high risk groups and the general population. Thus, these core groups must be targeted for intervention in all STI control programs. One such targeted intervention strategy which has been found to be effective in several countries is the Periodic Presumptive Treatment (PPT) of STIs. This involves periodic (usually monthly) administration of specific antibiotics (e.g. Azithromycin) to these core groups whether they have symptoms or not. This approach is considered cost effective when done in the short term and once STI prevalence is reduced, other approaches including socio-behavioural change strategies can be used to sustain the reduction.

3

Control and Prevention of Sexually Transmitted Infections

With the huge burden imposed by sexually transmitted infections (STIs) globally, it is essential that effective control and preventive measures are implemented in every country. The control interventional measures aim at achieving reduction in both the prevalence and incidence of STIs to acceptable level, and may be grouped into primary, secondary and other targeted prevention approaches. Globally, many of these interventional approaches have been used for a long time and there may be the need to adapt them to current socio-cultural and behavioural trends in other to make them more effective in application and outcome, within country specific contexts.

Primary prevention interventions

These are measures which mainly involve socio-behavioural change strategies using information, education and communication (IEC) tools or peer-led educational strategies. These aim at ensuring that people avoid what would put them at risk of getting an STI, thus reducing the incidence of STIs. These measures include education on risk elimination and risk reduction which may be carried out as mass campaigns or individualized education or counseling in various settings including the health care setting.

This approach may involve education on abstinence and the promotion of safer sex practices as espoused by the 'A, B, C' strategies thus:

- A: abstinence from sex
- B: being mutually faithful with an uninfected partner
- C: correct and consistent use of condoms

Depending on the target population (e.g. adolescents), various aspects of these measures are emphasized. These measures have their limitations for different groups but have proven to be very important components of all STI prevention interventions. These can help individuals particularly delay sexual debut and subsequent sexual activity, reduce number of sexual partners and adopt less risky sexual practices. Thus condom promotion including improved access and availability is very essential. More recently, the use of safe microbicides, is being promoted as a primary prevention measure for some STIs including HIV.

In addition to these, primary preventive measures include vaccinations for specific organisms. Human papillomavirus (HPV) and hepatitis B virus (HBV) vaccines are the main examples. The most widely available and used STI vaccine is the HBV vaccine which is part of childhood vaccines for most countries including Ghana. The different HPV vaccines targeting different genotypes of the virus, have been shown to be an essential primary prevention measure against genital warts and cervical cancer. These vaccines have been mostly available in developed countries but are in recent years becoming available for use in developing counties including Ghana. There is however no national policy on the universal application of these vaccines as part of the national immunization programme. The associated significant cost is also a barrier which must be addressed in resource-constrained setting.

Generally STI prevention and control interventions which focus on females are recommended as these empower them to have control over their sexual behaviours and practices. Hence the promotion of female condoms, vaginal microbicides and other pre-exposure prophylactic measures are considered important and invaluable in STI prevention and control. Overall the economic empowerment of women grants them power of choice and bargain and is therefore considered an important strategy when implemented with other interventions.

Secondary prevention interventions

These mainly involve screening to identify infected persons including asymptomatic carriers and managing them. This intervention can be done as community level screening for some STIs and also at facility level for vulnerable groups like pregnant women. In Ghana, pregnant women are routinely offered testing for syphilis, HBV and HIV during antenatal visits. Point of care (POC) tests with high sensitivity and specificity have improved coverage for this intervention. When linked with partner notification and management, this strategy can help reduce the prevalence of STIs in the particular geographical area by reducing the number of asymptomatic carriers. This leads to the break in the chain of transmission. It is important to also implement interventions which reduce mother-to-child transmission of STIs. Such measure have been developed particularly for Syphilis, HIV, and HBV.

This strategy will have better impact when it addresses issues like improving access to care and improving case management.

Targeted prevention interventions

High risk groups like sex workers (SWs) and men who have sex with men (MSM) require specific targeted interventions and thus are usually reached with screening activities and interventions like the Periodic Presumptive Treatment (PPT) (described in chapter 2) as a means of reducing STI prevalence and incidence in such high risk populations.

Challenges in STI control

An important challenge to STI control in recent times is the development of antimicrobial resistance by the pathogens. A typical example is *Neisseria gonorrhoeae* being resistant to common antibiotics such as penicillin and other commonly used ones. This then requires that antimicrobial susceptibility testing be done which is a challenge in most resource-constrained settings which have high gonorrhoea prevalence. Many of these countries have been unable to establish an *N. gonorrhoeae* surveillance programme. The World Health Organization (WHO) has attempted to deal with this challenge with the establishment of the gonococcal antimicrobial susceptibility programme (GASP).

In most countries particularly developing countries, there is lack of integration of STI related activities with different control programmes, with each implementing different parallel programmes. It is essential that efforts are made to integrate services and activities. Such integration with reproductive health and other services has proven beneficial in different settings. It helps to increase coverage and access.

In summary, to be effective, all STI prevention and control strategies must address the following:

- Reducing exposure.
- Reducing barriers to services.
- Promote services.
- Raising awareness in communities.
- Reaching out to those who would not normally access reproductive health services (e.g. males, adolescents and young people).

4

Gonorrhoea

Aetiology

Gonorrhoea is caused by the Gram-negative cocci *Neisseria gonorrhoea,* an obligate human pathogen transmitted mainly via sexual contact. The sexual contact could be through vaginal, oral or anal sex. The interaction between *N. gonorrhoea* and the host immune system ensures that, the host is unable to develop an immunological memory against the pathogen, hence re-infection may occur.

Epidemiology

The disease affects people of all ages, races, and socioeconomic status but adolescents and young adults are the highest risk group, with more than 80% of the reported cases each year occurring in the 15-29 age group. Individuals with unsafe sexual practices including having multiple sexual partners are at an increased risk, hence higher incidence among commercial sex workers. Transmission of *N. gonorrhoea* is very efficient. In fact, women run a 60-90% chance of contracting the disease after just one sexual encounter with an infected sexual partner. Majority (about 80%) of women remain asymptomatic for a long time and thus become a continuous source (reservoirs) of transmission to sexual partners. Babies are also infected usually during delivery by an untreated infected mother, resulting in infection of the eyes and leading to ophthalmia neonatorum. In addition, infection of the eyes of babies can be through contact with contaminated fingers of infected persons.

Clinical presentation

The incubation period is usually 2-10 days with men in particular becoming symptomatic with urethral discharge and associated dysuria and frequency of urination. Symptomatic women complain of vaginal discharge with or without dysuria and with or without lower abdominal pain depending on the severity of the condition. Mainly, women also commonly have co-infection with other organisms particularly Chlamydia infection. Many people with gonococcal proctitis are asymptomatic. When symptoms occur, they commonly include rectal pain or itching, a rectal discharge, rectal bleeding and/or a persistent urge to move the bowels. This is most often seen in Men who have Sex with Men (MSM) but can be seen in women who engage in anal sex. In new-borns, symptoms appear one to four days after birth and can affect one or both eyes. Symptoms include redness of the eyes, swelling of the eyelids, photophobia and eye discharge due to the conjunctivitis. The discharge in all these cases is usually muco-purulent or purulent. If gonorrhoea spreads through the bloodstream (septicaemia), it may spread to various organs and tissues with resultant symptoms such as fever, pain, swelling in one or several joints (arthritis), and a characteristic rash. Complications of untreated gonorrhoea include:

- Infertility in women: Untreated gonorrhoea can spread into the uterus and fallopian tubes, causing pelvic inflammatory disease (PID), which may result in scarring of the tubes, greater risk of pregnancy complications (ectopic pregnancy) and infertility. Infertility in men: Men with untreated gonorrhoea can experience epididymo-orchitis which when left untreated, may lead to infertility by affecting sperm production and quality.

- Disseminated gonococcal infection (DGI): this can be a serious complication resulting in death if not treated quickly. The inflammatory condition of the joins (arthritis) may have long term sequelae among survivors. It is seen often in women who might have asymptomatic genital infection.

- Complications in babies: Ophthalmia neonatorum can result in blindness if not treated promptly due to corneal damage.

- Peri-hepatitis (Curtis-Fitz-Hugh Syndrome): this can occur in both males and females. In this condition, inflammation involving the capsule of the liver results in formation of adhesions.

Diagnosis

Gonorrhoea can be diagnosed using the syndromic, clinical or aetiologic approaches described in chapter two. In all cases a thorough history taking is essential to aid diagnosis. This must be followed by a detailed physical examination, which may require passing vaginal speculum to visualize the cervix and also proctoscope for examination of the rectum. Standard algorithms may be used per the Syndromic protocols to arrive at a diagnosis.

It is increasingly essential to have an aetiological diagnosis of gonorrhoea, requiring the identification of the causative agent from clinical samples (swabs from vaginal, urethral, rectal or eyes discharges). These swabs must be processed rapidly as *N. gonorrhoea* is susceptible to drying. Microscopy from smears is about 85% sensitive (from urethral discharge) as it shows the typically intracellular kidney-shaped diplococci. Sensitivity is lower in samples taken from the oral cavity and also from vaginal discharge. Due to the appearance of drug resistance strains, it has become necessary to culture samples and isolate *N. gonorrhoea* for drug sensitivity testing in most parts of the world. This is very necessary especially when the person does not respond to initial treatment or become symptomatic soon after treatment.

The organism is fastidious requiring nutrient supplementation to grow hence are usually isolated on Thayer-Martin agar (or VPN agar) which contains antibiotics (Vancomycin, Colistin, Nystatin and Trimethoprim) and nutrients that facilitate the growth of Neisseria species while inhibiting the growth of contaminating bacteria and fungi. Other such specialized media are available for isolation of *N. gonorrhoea.* Identification tests include the oxidase test (N. gonorrhoea are oxidase positive) and the carbohydrates utilization test (N. gonorrhoea utilizes only glucose).

Nucleic acid amplification tests (NAATs) are also available for identification from samples and these methods are increasingly becoming essential for screening.

NAATs detect gonococcal DNA in samples including urine. These tests have been reported to have different sensitivity and specificity values based on the clinical sample used for screening.

Treatment, Prevention and Control

Gonorrhoea is usually treated under the syndromic management approach in many countries including Ghana with a combination of drugs to cover for all possible causes of genital discharge syndrome. Gonorrhoea has become more difficult and expensive to treat since the 1970s, due to the increased resistance of gonorrhoea to common antibiotics. The spread of such drug resistant strains has been increasing steadily and hence is a challenge in the treatment and control of gonorrhoea globally.

Uncomplicated gonorrhoea is easy to treat and should usually respond to a single dose therapy with the right antibiotic. Medications used to treat gonorrhoea include Ceftriaxone, Cefixime, Spectinomycin, and Ciprofloxacin. The commonest protocol is:

- I.M. Ceftriaxone 250mg stat

  OR

- Tab Ciprofloxacin 500 mg stat (contraindicated in pregnancy)

  OR

- Tab Cefixime 400mg stat

  OR

- Tab Azithromycin 2g stat

  OR

- IM Spectinomycin 2g stat

In countries with limited data on the drug susceptibility pattern, WHO recommends dual therapy involving either 250mg IM Ceftriaxone or oral Cefixime 400 mg stat plus oral azithromycin 1g stat. For the management of dessemnated gonococcal infections, IM or IV Ceftriaxone 1g daily for 7 days or IM Spectinomycin 2g 12 hrly for 7 days is recommended. The duration of treatment for other complicated forms like gonococcal meningitis and endocarditis have to be extened to up to 4 weeks.

If re-infection is suspected after initial treatment, it is recommended that treatment is repeated according to the protocol but better still efforts be made to obtain antimicrobial susceptibility profile of the isolate to guide treatment. This is even more essential when treatment failure is suspected.

The drug choice is also influenced by breastfeeding or pregnancy status of women in which case Ciprofloxacin is not used. All sexual partner(s) during the time of infection, even if those partners do not show symptoms, need to be notified and treated.

Ophthalmia neonatorum can be treated with I.M. Ceftriaxone 50mg/kg (maximum 125mg) stat or IM Spectinomycin 25mg/kg (maximum 75mg) stat.

Additionally the mother and her partner must both be treated for Gonorrhoea.

As a preventive measure the cleaning of the eyes and the application of 1% tetracycline ointment or 1% silver nitrate solution to the eyes of babies at birth is to be undertaken routinely.

5

Sexually Transmitted Chlamydia Infections

Aetiology

Chlamydiae trachomatis (C. trachomatis) belongs to the family *Chlamydiaceae,* an obligate, aerobic, non-motile, and an intracellular bacteria. It has a cytoplasmic membrane and outer membrane but, it lacks a peptidoglycan cell wall. There are many serovars of *C. trachomatis* and these include *C. trachomatis serovars* D-K and *Lymphogranuloma venereum* (LGV) serovars L1, L2 and L3 which are sexually transmitted.

Epidemiology

C. trachomatis infections occur worldwide and is the leading cause of bacterial genital infections among women. Women often get repeated chlamydia genital infections in their life time. LGV is endemic in developing countries in Africa, South America, Asia and the Caribbean. The greatest risk factors for infection are age and sex, where rates of infection are observed to be highest amongst females 15-24 years of age, and males 20-24 years. However, there have been an increasing number of cases in the developed world among men who have sex with men (MSMs). Chlamydia is a significant public health problem because untreated chlamydia may lead to pelvic inflammatory disease, subfertility and poor reproductive outcomes in some women. Chlamydia also facilitates the transmission of HIV. Although inexpensive and effective treatment is available, control of chlamydia is challenging since most people are asymptomatic. Transmission to neonates occur during birth resulting in conjunctivitis.

LGV can be transmitted through vaginal, anal or oral sexual contact. Genital infections are transmitted sexually through direct genital-genital or genital-anal contact. Vertical transmission to new-borns can also occur, most commonly during passage through the birth canal.

Clinical presentation

Chlamydia STI is known as a "silent" disease because about 75 percent of infected women and at least half of infected men have no symptoms. Presentation is similar to that of gonorrhoea. Thus clinical diagnosis has very low sensitivity and specificity. Incubation period ranges from a week to few months.

- Genital infections: *C. trachomatis* may cause infection and inflammation of the reproductive tract, urethritis, proctitis, and epididymitis in men and urethritis, endometritis, salpingitis, and cervicitis in women. Infections may mostly be asymptomatic. Symptomatic female patients often experience pelvic pain, burning urination, pain during sex and abnormal vaginal bleeding, with inflammation of the endocervical columnar epithelium. Symptomatic male patients often experience urethral discharge, dysuria, and painful swelling in the testicles. Untreated infection can result in long-term sequelae such as pelvic inflammatory disease (PID) and infertility in females, epididymitis and infertility in males, and reactive arthritis

(Reiter's syndrome) and perihepatitis (Fitz-Hugh-Curtis syndrome) in both males and females. The infection can also be passed to newborns during childbirth resulting in conjunctivitis or pneumonia. Infection may also result in pregnancy complications, such as abortion, stillbirth, prematurity, and intrauterine foetal infections. Untreated infections can increase vulnerability to HIV infection. Both men and women can have infection with Chlamydia in the rectum if they have anal sex and this may cause rectal discharge or discomfort, but often no symptoms occur.

- Neonatal conjunctivitis: seen in neonates within 2 weeks after delivery. The eyelids are swollen, shut and have purulent discharge. Complications include blindness and also pneumonia.

- *Lymphogranuloma venereum (LGV):* This condition is caused by different serological variants (serovars L1, L2, and L3,) of Chlamydia and infection first presents as genital ulcers followed by lymphadenopathy presenting as inguinal buboes. Symptoms include chills, headache, myalgia, and arthralgia. Infection can further spread into the eyes, central nervous system, heart and lungs. Untreated LGV can result in lymphatic obstruction and elephantiasis of genitalia.

Laboratory Diagnosis

Chlamydiae are intracellular organisms, and it is therefore essential to obtain host cells with the clinical sample to ensure yield of organisms. The sensitivity and specificity of any test for *Chlamydia trachomatis,* is highly dependent on sampling and adequacy of the sample obtained. In women, the endocervix is most commonly targeted for obtaining samples for culture, by using either a swab or a cytologic brush. Adequate sample can be obtained using Dacron, cotton, rayon or calcium alginate-tipped swabs with plastic shafts. Sampling is performed by inserting the swab approximately 1-2 cm into the cervical os, rotating it, and keeping it in situ for some seconds before withdrawing it.

In male patients, the anterior urethra is the site of choice for optimal sampling, especially for culture purposes. A dry swab is inserted 3 to 4 cm past the meatal opening of the urethra, rotated and removed. It is important to note that urination should best be avoided for at least 1 hour prior to sampling, as this significantly reduces the yield of cells obtained during sampling. A urine sample may also be required only for males. A swab is used to collect cells from the rectum and throat, and these swabs are routinely recommended for persons engaging in anal or oral sex. For LGV, sampling can be in the form of swabs from ulcers, saline aspirates from the biopsies. To ensure adequacy of samples taken from deep-seated ulcers in the rectum, these biopsies may be best performed under direct vision through proctoscopy.

In cases of conjunctivitis, a swab is used to collect epithelial cells from the palpebral conjunctival surface on the eye.

Tissue culture is required for isolating the bacteria and it requires embryonated egg of a hen or animal cell lines. This technique therefore is not usually done. Cell lines available for use including McCoy cells and HeLa 229 cells. These methods are expensive and labour intensive. The sensitivity of culture methods range between 70-85% depending on the specific method and other factors.

Direct fluorescent test (DFA) has remained one of the useful methods for detecting Chlamydia in clinical samples. It is simple, rapid and involved identification of the elementary bodies in smears after staining. It involves using monoclonal antibodies and fluorescein stain resulting in the elementary bodies appearing as apple green particles. Sensitivity and specificity ranges between 80-99% compared with culture. Diagnosis is also possible through ELISA which is available but with sensitivity and specificity around 60-90% and hence not very often used in clinical care.

Nucleic acid amplification tests are commercially available and are commonly used in developed countries. These have better specificity and sensitivity but sensitivity is said to be reduced in countries with low prevalence of infection. PCR assays are available with many different types and assays but very much limited to resource rich countries.

Thus, diagnosis of Chlamydia infection in routine patient care is limited in Ghana and confirmation of infection is seen mostly in scientific research but not in clinical care. In patient care, chlamydia infections are diagnosed with the vaginal or urethral discharge syndromes and managed according to the flow charts at most health service delivery points.

Treatment

The treatment of *C. trachomatis* infection depends on the site of the infection, the age of the patient, and whether the infection is complicated or uncomplicated. Treatment also differs during pregnancy. Chlamydia can be easily treated and cured with antibiotics. Patients are advised to abstain from sexual intercourse for seven days after treatment initiation.

The recommended and the most commonly used treatment options are:

- A single dose of Azithromycin 1g (preferred in pregnancy); OR
- Cap Doxycycline 100mg twice daily for 7 days.

  Alternatives include:

- Tab Erythromycin 500mg 6hourly for 7 days
- Levofloxacin or Ofloxacin 200mg twice a day for 7 days.

Doxycycline, Tetracycline, Levofloxacin, Ciprofloxacin and Ofloxacin, are contraindicated in pregnant and lactating mothers.

Babies with Chlamydial conjunctivitis are treated with oral Azithromycin 20mg/kg daily for 3 days;

OR

Oral Erythromycin 50mg/kg a day in four divided doses for 14 days.

The recommended medical treatment for LGV involves one of the following antibiotic regimens:

- Cap Doxycycline 100mg twice a day for 21 days (preferred)
  OR
- Oral Azithromycin 1g weekly for 3 weeks
  OR
- Tab Erythromycin 500mg 6hourly for 14 days

Inguinal buboes could be drained using wide bore needle through the surrounding healthy skin but incision and drainage directly should not be done.

Prevention and control

Primary prevention starts with changing sexual behaviours that increase the risk of contracting the infection. Annual screening for chlamydial infection in all sexually active women 24 years and younger, and in women older than 24 years who are at risk of STDs (e.g., have a new sex partner, have a history of multiple sex partners) is a necessary preventive and control tool where feasible. Additionally, there should be a routine case surveillance, accurate chlamydia diagnostic services, clinical services, and patient and partner management services.The use of condom during each sexual contact helps reduce infection. Thus, condoms used properly during every sexual encounter will reduce chlamydia infection but will not eliminate the risk of infection. Contact tracing and treat- ment is essential.

Prevention of neonatal conjunctivitis requires that immediately following delivery, baby's eyes are cleaned and 1% tetracycline ointment or 1% Silver Nitrate solution is applied.

6

Syphilis

Aetiology

Syphilis is a systemic disease caused by the *Treponema pallidum,* a spirochaete. *T. pallidum,* was identified in 1905 and its associate disease remains an important public health problem especially in developing countries including Ghana. Its link with HIV infection also makes this condition very important. It has been proven that syphilis and its associated genital ulcer, increases the risk of HIV transmission and acquisition.

Epidemiology

The infection can be classified as congenital (transmitted from mother to child in utero) or acquired primarily through sex or other means including transfusion of contaminated blood. The risk of foetal infection heightens with increasing gestational age, with the highest risk (90%) occurring when a woman has primary syphilis during late pregnant. In Ghana the prevalence of syphilis has continued to reduce in the past years due to introduction of specific protocols. These have included the need to screen all pregnant women and treat immediately and link to partner notification and screening. The Central Region of Ghana has for the past decade or more been the region with the highest prevalence of syphilis amongst pregnant women in the country. It is expected that increased screening and treatment will continue to reduce the prevalence of Syphilis.

Clinical presentation

Primary syphilis

The first stage of syphilis known as primary syphilis is characterized by the appearance of an ulcer or chancre at the site of infection or inoculation. This ulcer is mostly single, painless, indurated with a clear base and well-defined edges. It is usually associated with a painless lymphadenopathy. The chancre heals spontaneously within 2-6 weeks without scaring and hence may go unnoticed to the infected person. This lesion could also occur in the anus or rectum and other extragenital sites.

Secondary syphilis

Manifestations of this stage include the appearance of a generalized skin rash, mucocutaneous lesions and generalized lymphadenopathy. The rash is usually macular at the beginning and may become maculopapular with time. It may occur about 2 months after the appearance of the primary chancre. It can spread all over the body, or appear in patches, and it is often seen on the palms of the hands and soles of the feet. There may be flat, wart-like growths on the vulva in women and around the anus in both men and women. This stage is highly infectious. The lesions may disappear spontaneously in about 2-3 months.

Latent syphilis

Early latent syphilis

This stage is seen usually within 2 years of infection. Mostly there are no clinical evidence of treponemal infection. Sometimes, there are development of lesions on the body which can appear anywhere. In women, they are found mainly on the vulva, the clitoris, cervix, and around the opening of the urethra, and the anus. In men, they appear mainly around the opening of the urethra, on the penis and foreskin, and around the anus.

Tertiary or late latent syphilis

This usually implies an infection lasting decade(s) in duration. This may, after many years, start to cause serious damage to the heart, brain, bones and nervous system. Slowly progressive, destructive inflammatory lesions develop and the 3 most common presentations are Neurosyphilis, Cardiovascular syphilis and Gummatous syphilis.

Congenital syphilis

This usually results in miscarriages and stillbirths as a consequence. Infected babies who are born without obvious symptoms may still develop early signs within 2 years of age. These signs include skin and subcutaneous tissue manifestations. They may experience failure to thrive, develop chorioretinitis and other related problems. Late manifestations occurring after 2 years of age include Hutchinson's teeth, Glaucoma, Mental retardation, blindness, deafness and others.

Diagnosis

Evaluation starts with a detailed history including sexual history, followed by thorough physical examination. Under the syndromic approach, it is classified under the genital ulcer syndromes. Blood samples are commonly used for laboratory testing for syphilis, but cerebrospinal fluid could be used in neurosyphilis.

Serology is the main method used. are two main types of syphilis serological tests:

- Non treponemal tests (non-specific antibody tests): The common tests used are the Rapid Plasma Reagin (RPR) and the Venereal Disease Research Laboratory (VDRL) tests. The disadvantage of these tests is the false positive results in conditions like leprosy, yaws, connective tissue diseases and even some viral and parasitic infections. In addition, they may give false negative results in the late stages.

- Treponemal test (specific antibody tests): Commonly Treponema Pallidum Heam Agglutination (TPHA) and the Fluorescent Treponemal Antibody Absorption (FTA) tests. They have the limitation of remaining positive after treatment.

Rapid tests are available and currently done on the spot in consultation rooms by health workers, with results being made available within 15-20 minutes. These are used in antenatal clinics in Ghana by midwives for routine testing of all pregnant women.

Treatment, Prevention and Control

Penicillin is the most common treatment for syphilis, but there are alternative antibiotics that can be used. The recommended treatment is Benzathine Penicillin G 2.4 million units stat for primary and secondary stages in adolescents and adults including pregnant women. The alternative is IM procaine benzyl penicillin 1.2 million IU daily for 10-14 days.

Alternatives to Penicillin include:

- Cap Doxycycline 100mg 12 hourly for 14 days (should not be used for pregnant women).
  OR
- I.M. Ceftriaxone 1g once daily for 10–14 days.
- Tab Azithromycin 2g once.

Latent and tertiary stages require longer duration of treatment. The recommendation for latent syphilis is Benzathine Penicillin G 2.4 million units once a week for 3 consecutive weeks or IM procaine benzyl penicillin 1.2 million IU daily for 20 days. This is recommended also for cases where the stage of syphilis cannot be determined. Neurosyphilis requires even longer duration of treatment.

Babies born to positive mothers who were not treated, were treated with alternatives to Penicillin or were treated less than 30 days before delivery require treatment. The recommendations include:

1. Aqueous benzyl penicillin 100,000-150,000 U/kg/day IV for 10-15 days.

2. Procaine penicillin 50,000 U/kg/day as a single dose IV for 10-15 days.

All other infants born to infected mothers but who do not meet the criteria for treatment must be monitored.

Some people get a reaction known as the Jarisch-Herx-Heimer reaction to treatment. This is a flu-like illness with high temperature, headache and aches and pains in the muscles and joints. This usually starts within 4–6 hours after treatment and lasts for up to 24 hours. It is thought to be caused by the release of toxins into the bloodstream when the bacteria die. This may be treated with oral prednisolone. Control of syphilis is based on safer sex practices, early diagnosis and treatment.

7

Chancroid

Aetiology

Chancroid is a sexually transmitted infection (STI) caused by *Haemophilus ducreyi,* a Gram negative coccobacillus. It presents as an acute bacterial infection localized in the genital area and characterized clinically by single or multiple painful, necrotizing ulcers, frequently accompanied by painful swelling and/or suppuration of regional lymph nodes.

Epidemiology

A break in the skin around the genitalia during intercourse is usually required for sexual transmission to occur. It is more common in tropical regions. The global incidence has decreased significantly over the years but regions which mainly have cases include Africa, Asia, Central and South America.

Clinical presentation

Chancroid was one of the causes of genital ulcer disease (GUD) in many parts of the world but its incidence has now decreased markedly. It is characterized by anogenital ulceration and lymphadenitis with progression to bubo formation. The usual incubation period is 4-10 days and there are no prodromal symptoms. A chancroid lesion starts as a tender papule that develops into a pustule and which may result in a painful necrotizing genital ulcer or soft chancre. Classically, ulcers have a ragged undermined edge with a grey or yellow base that bleeds when touched. The usual sites of infection are, in men, the prepuce, coronal sulcus, frenulum and glans and in women, the labia minora and fourchette. Ulcers of the vaginal wall and cervix are uncommon. Extra-genital lesions caused by *H. ducreyi* are rare but have been reported on the fingers, breasts and inner thighs. *H. ducreyi* does not disseminate systemically and its asymptomatic carriage is rare.

Painful inguinal lymphadenopathy is found in about half of the cases presented in males but less in women. These lymph glands may develop into buboes that should be managed by aspiration rather than incision and drainage. Fluctuant buboes may rupture spontaneously causing delayed healing. Complications are mostly seen in men and may include phimosis and partial loss of tissue particularly on the glans penis. Healed ulcers may result in tissue contraction and predispose to mucosal breaks and bleeding that might increase the risk of HIV transmission during sexual intercourse.

Diagnosis

Following a detailed history and physical examination, a clinical or syndromic diagnosis could be made. Under the syndromic approach, it is diagnosed as part of the painful genital ulcer syndrome. Aetiological diagnosis involves the identification of *H. ducreyi* in the laboratory. This is difficult because the organism is very fastidious.

Microscopy of a Gram stained smear (or other stains) of material from the ulcer base or of pus aspirate from the bubo may show characteristic Gramnegative cocco-bacilli, with occasional characteristic chaining. Culture of material obtained from the base or edges of the ulcer, or pus aspirated from the bubo can be done. Culture media include Mueller-Hinton agar enriched with 5% heated horse blood to provide the factor X (haemin) required and other enriched media. Since *H ducreyi* is a fastidious organism, specimens should be plated out directly at the clinic or sent rapidly (within 4 hours) to the laboratory and may require transport media e.g. Amie's or Stuart's medium. In the laboratory, plates should preferably be incubated at 33°C in a humid atmosphere containing 5% CO_2 for between 3 -7 days. Multiple PCR assays have also been developed for the simultaneous amplification of DNA targets from *H. ducreyi, T. palladium* and *HSV types* 1 and 2. These assays improve the sensitivity compared with culture methods.

Treatment, Prevention and Control

Treatment of Chancroid should successful cure infection, resolve clinical symptoms, and prevent transmission to sexual partners. Considerations for drug choice include pregnancy and history of drug allergies. Drugs include:

- Azithromycin 1g orally stat
  OR
- I. M. Ceftriaxone 250 mg stat
  OR
- Ciprofloxacin 500 mg orally 12 hourly for 3 days
  OR
- Erythromycin 500 mg orally 6 hourly for 7 days

Supportive therapy may include drainage of fluctuant buboes using a large bore needle inserted through healthy skin and managing the ulcer. All sexual contacts of a person with Chancroid (contact within 10 days preceding the development of symptoms) should be contacted and offered antibiotic treatment whether they are symptomatic or not. In addition, it is essential to offer HIV testing and counseling for all cases of Chancroid because of the increased risk of acquisition and transmission. These patients should also be screened for syphilis and if available Herpes simplex virus.

8

Donovanosis

Aetiology

Donovanosis (Granuloma Inguinale), is a chronic cause of genital ulceration caused by *Klebsiella granulomatis* formerly called *Calymmatobacterium granulomatis.* The condition has often been described in recent times by medical scientists as forgotten or overlooked. Interest in donovanosis waned and the disease attracted little attention following the discovery of antibiotics until the late 1980s when genital ulcers were identified as a significant co-factor in facilitating HIV transmission.

Epidemiology

Donovanosis has a curious geographical distribution with "hotspots" in Papua New Guinea, parts of India and Brazil. Sporadic cases are reported elsewhere in Southern Africa, the West Indies, and South America.

Clinical presentation

Donovanosis usually causes genital ulcerations that bleeds easily to the touch and are usually painless. The incubation period is uncertain. Estimates are very varied with ranges between 1–360 days, 3–40 days, 14–28 days, etc. Infection usually starts as a firm papule or subcutaneous nodule that ulcerates. Classically there are four types of donovanosis:

- Ulcero-granulomatous type: the commonest type presenting as beefy red, non-tender ulcers that bleed easily to touch and may become quite extensive if left untreated
- Hypertrophic or verrucous ulcer: there is a growth usually with an irregular edge
- Necrotic types: foul smelling deep ulcers with extensive tissue destruction.
- Sclerotic, or cicatricial lesion with fibrous and scar tissue formation.

The anatomical areas affected most frequently in men, are the coronal sulcus, sub-preputial region, and anus. In women it affects the labia minora, fourchette, and occasionally the cervix and upper genital tract. Ulcers are more common in uncircumcised men with poor standards of genital hygiene. Extragenital lesions account for 6% of cases and sites of infection include lip, gums, cheek, palate, pharynx, neck, nose, larynx, and chest. Rarely, disseminated donovanosis with spread to bone and liver may occur and is usually associated with pregnancy and cervical infection. However, ulcers may sometimes be difficult to differentiate from primary syphilitic chancres, condylomata lata of secondary syphilis, chancroid, and large HIV associated herpes ulcers. Donovanosis associated pseudo-elephantiasis may mimic Lymphogranuloma venereum (LGV). Donovanosis is often long standing and the possibility of dual infection with one or other of the classic causes of genital ulcer disease (GUD) should always be considered. Extragenital lesions may present atypically often leading to protracted delay in the diagnosis.

Diagnosis

Confirmation is by the identification of typical intra-cellular donovanosis bodies within large mononuclear cells, either in smears obtained directly from tissue or biopsy samples. These characteristic cells are 25–90 μm in diameter while the donovanosis bodies are 0.5– 0.7 by 1–1.5 μm and may or may not be capsulated. The following are recommended diagnostic tests:

- Staining by a slow overnight Giemsa method or Leishman's or Wright's stain. Pieces of tissue obtained by using forceps and scalpel from the advancing surface of the ulcer can be crushed between two slides, taking care not to cause drying of the specimen by prolonged spreading. Alternatively, the clean undersurface of the tissue can be smeared along a glass slide. If donovanosis is considered likely but multiple swabs are taken from ulcers to detect other potential pathogens, it is important that the smear for Donovan bodies is taken first so that adequate material can be obtained from the surface of the ulcer. Clearly, most ulcers will be dry after a few swabs have been taken and it will then be difficult to demonstrate Donovan bodies in superficial tissue smears. Specimens from sites just below the surface of the ulcer are more likely to yield positive results than those from superficial tissue. If time allows, biopsy, fixing in formaldehyde, embedding in paraffin and slow, overnight, Giemsa should provide optimal results.

- Biopsies can be done under local anaesthetic and examined by histology. The best stains to use are either Giemsa or silver rather than haematoxylin and eosin. Histological changes of donovanosis usually show epithelial proliferation and a heavy inflammatory infiltrate of plasma cells, neutrophils, and few lymphocytes. Biopsy is usually required to confirm the diagnosis for the necrotic and sclerotic variants and sometimes for hypertrophic lesions.

- Polymerase chain reaction (PCR) - Although these techniques have been reported, the process is still really only available as a research tool and requires further evaluation.

- Serology - An indirect immunofluorescent technique has been developed using thin sections of donovanosis lesions as a source of antigen with good results for established lesions but with a low sensitivity for early infection. While the test might be useful in population studies in endemic areas, it is not accurate enough at the individual level to be acceptable for confirmatory diagnosis.

The diagnosis of donovanosis, particularly when associated with extragenital lesions, is often missed in non-endemic areas because it is not suspected. In areas where the condition is well known and described, a high index of clinical suspicion should be maintained for unusual manifestations of genital ulcers and other skin lesions appearing in extragenital sites.

There is a dilemma in recommending optimal treatment for donovanosis depending on whether or not strict syndromic guidelines for GUD are recommended and adhered to. In most areas where donovanosis is found, chancroid is also prevalent and has a higher incidence.

Syndromic protocols recommend treatment for syphilis and Chancroid too.

Treatment, Prevention and Control

Currently, Azithromycin is probably the best drug available for donovanosis in that, it can be given intermittently, the total pill count is low, directly observed therapy is possible, and treatment can usually be stopped before ulcers have healed completely. WHO guidelines recommend Azithromycin 1g immediately then 500mg daily but does not state the duration of therapy and instead state that it be continued until the patient is completely cured. Other antibiotics that may be effective if given for 3 weeks or until ulcers have healed fully include Cotrimoxazole 160/800mg twice daily, Ciprofloxacin 750mg twice daily, Doxycycline 100mg twice daily or Gentamicin 1mg/kg three times daily, intramuscularly or intravenously if no response is observed in the first few days with other regimens.

There is a high tendency for recurrence despite good initial responses to treatment. Epidemiological treatment can be considered in the absence of signs and symptoms in sexual partners of index cases. Female partners should be examined and a speculum examination included to detect possible cervical infection.

9

Genital Herpes

Aetiology

Genital herpes is one of the most common sexually transmitted infections (STIs). It is best known for the sores and blisters it causes. Genital herpes is usually caused by Herpes simplex virus (HSV) type-2 though type 1 strains have also been increasingly identified in the genital tract. Herpes viruses are a large family of microorganisms that belong to a family known as herpesviridae. All are double stranded DNA enveloped viruses capable of latency. HSV is a nuclear replicating, icosahedral shaped virus.

Epidemiology

HSV-1 and HSV-2 occur worldwide and have no seasonal variation. Most human beings (about 90% of adults) have been infected and harbour latent virus that can reactivate. Hence, there is a vast HSV reservoir for transmission to susceptible individuals. Transmission predominantly occurs during anogenital contact. Some transmission occurs during oro-genital contact. Infections transmitted from the mouth to the anogenital area are usually type 1. An infection by one type at one mucosal site does not protect against acquisition at another mucosal site, but the signs and symptoms are then much less severe. Transmission from an infected mother to her baby rarely occurs via the placenta, as mother-to-child transmission mostly occur during labor and delivery, or after birth through indirect contact with the mother's infected secretions. HSV-2 sero-prevalence in sub-Saharan Africa is among the highest in the world, sometimes reaching >80% in women and men aged >35 years. A central public health problem of genital herpes is the high proportion of genital HSV infections that are unrecognized by both patients and clinicians.

Clinical Presentation

Most people with genital herpes have no symptoms or do not notice them. Symptoms may last several weeks, go away and recur later. The frequency and severity of symptoms vary from person to person. Primary infection has an incubation period between 2-15 days. The most common symptom is a cluster of vesicles that appear on the penis, vagina, cervix, anus, buttocks or (rarely) elsewhere on the body. They start as small pimples or blisters that soon become open, painful shallow ulcers. The sores usually heal within 2-4 weeks. Associated symptoms may include pain or discomfort around the genitals, buttocks or legs, swollen lymph nodes in the groin, burning sensation while urinating, and flu-like symptoms (fever, chills , headache or body aches). These symptoms are usually more severe during primary episodes than during recurrence.

After the first episode, the virus becomes latent in the dorsal root ganglia. Later on, the virus can reactivate and cause sores. During recurrence, the ulcers usually heal sooner and do not feel as painful as the first episode. In general, recurrences are most common in the first year after infection. Genital herpes caused by HSV-2 is much more likely to recur than genital herpes caused by HSV-1. Recurrences may be more frequent for people with weakened immune systems especially HIV/AIDS clients. Although a person may not know what triggered a recurrence, the patient may notice warning signs. These signs often include itching, tingling, numbness or tenderness where the lesions will appear. Sometimes there can be pain near the buttocks, back of legs or lower back. The warning signs may start a few hours to a day before the vesicles appear. Lesions can re-appear anywhere on or near the genitals, often at the same place as before. In some cases, the virus can reactivate without causing usual symptoms like blisters, itching or pain. This is called "asymptomatic shedding" or "subclinical shedding" and is most frequent in the first year of infection.

Complications of HSV infection may include aseptic meningitis and urinary retention due to autonomic neuropathy. Genital herpes also increases the risk of HIV transmission and acquisition.

Neonatal herpes, though rare, has a high mortality and morbidity rate. The risk is highest in mothers who develop primary infection close to delivery since these babies will acquire the virus in the absence of any protecting antibodies. These neonates within about a week may develop pneumonias, encephalitis or meningitis. It is essential that antiviral treatment is initiated early in order to reduce the rate of mortality and morbidity.

Diagnosis

The diagnosis of HSV infections is usually based on clinical presentation of the classical symptoms and history of recurrence. Syndromic diagnosis identifies it under genital ulcer syndrome based on clinical symptoms and signs. The methods available for laboratory tests to diagnose HSV infections include viral identification test (VIT), viral culture (tissue culture) and serologic test (antigen detection tests). Sample collection usually involves a cotton swab being used to collect some of the fluid in blisters or ulcer. These samples might require specific transport medium or temperature requirements to improve sensitivity. Molecular tests are used to detect the DNA through various PCR methods. Serological tests can usually detect herpes antibodies 4 – 6 weeks after infection but are not generally used.

Treatment, Prevention and Control

There is need to keep the ulcer clean to avoid super bacterial infection. Oral antiviral agents are effective in many ways for almost all HSV infected patients. Topical antiviral agents have limited efficacy in acute infections and have not shown efficacy in recurrences and there-fore are not recommended. Valaciclovir, Famciclovir, and Acyclovir can be used to treat herpes infections and also reduce infectivity. For first episodes recommended drug therapy for all patients including HIV infected pa-tients include:

- Tab Acyclovir 200mg five times a day for 10 days, OR
- Tab Acyclovir 400mg 8 hourly for 10 days, OR
- Famciclovir 250mg three times a day for 7 to 10 days,

OR

- Valaciclovir 500mg twice a day for 7 to 10 days.

Recurrence usually do not require treatment but when severe, these same drugs could be used but usually for 5 days duration of treatment. These drugs can speed the healing of sores during an outbreak. When taken daily, they can also reduce the number of episodes of recurrence and sometimes stop them altogether. This is called "suppressive therapy". Few patients may need to be on Acyclovir 400mg daily or valaciclovir 500mg daily or famciclovir 250mg daily in order to suppress frequent recurrence (4-6 episodes per year). This may especially be needed for HIV positive patients in which case the options are acyclovir 400mg 12 hourly or famciclovir 500mg 12 hourly or valaciclovir 500mg daily.

Safe sex practices including condom use reduces the risk of transmission. But condom usage does not completely eliminate the risk. Washing of hands with soap and water after any possible contact with lesions is very necessary. This practice reduces the risk of re-infection or passing the virus to someone else.

Genital herpes frequently causes psychological distress in people who know they are infected. Patients diagnosed with genital HSV infection usually have many questions and concerns. There is considerable shame, embarrassment, and stigma associated with having herpes. For many patients, the psychological impact is far more severe than the physical consequences of the disease.

10

Anogenital Warts

Aetiology

Genital warts are small fleshy growths, bumps or skin changes that appear on or around the genital or peri-anal area. They are caused by the *Human papillomavirus* (HPV), the most common sexually transmitted infection (STI) globally. Different HPV strains usually affect different parts of the body, including the hands and feet. There are about 40 different types of HPV that can affect the anogenital area. These are further grouped as high risk (hr-HPV) or low risk (lr-HPV) based on their ability to persist and cause cervical cancer in women. Anogenital warts are caused by the low risk types. Around 90% of all cases of anogenital warts are caused by two lr-HPV types 6 and type 11.

Epidemiology

HPV is globally distributed but with a high burden in Sub Saharan Africa. HPV is the most common STI and infection is acquired early in sexual history. Factors affecting the risk of getting HPV infection and developing the associated clinical conditions include age, age at first sexual intercourse, life time number of sexual partners, hormonal contraceptive usage, history of smoking etc. There is a high burden of anogenital warts among Men who have Sex with Men (MSM). Transmission in mainly through sexual contact but can also be transmitted through other direct contact.

Clinical presentation

Most people who have an HPV infection will not develop any visible warts. If genital warts do appear, it can be several weeks, months or even years after infection with the virus. The warts may appear as small, fleshy growths, bumps or skin changes anywhere on the genitals or around the anus. In some cases, the warts are so small they are difficult to notice. They can be as small as 1-5mm in diameter, but can also grow or spread into large masses in the genital or anal area. In some cases they look like small stalks. They may be hard ("keratinized") or soft. A person can have a single wart or clusters of multiple warts that grow together to form a kind of "cauliflower" appearance. They are usually painless and do not pose a serious threat to health. But they can be unpleasant to look at and cause psychological distress. Warts can become itchy and inflamed. If a wart becomes inflamed, it leads to bleeding from the urethra, vagina or anus. In addition, warts in the urethral meatus may affect the flow of urine. The most common places for genital warts to develop in women are:

- around the vulva
- on the cervix
- on the walls of the vagina
- around or inside the anus

The most common places for genital warts to develop in men are:

- anywhere on the penis
- on the scrotum
- at the urethral meatus
- around or inside the anus

Diagnosis

The diagnosis of genital warts is most often made clin-ically, but may require confirmation by biopsy in some cases. Smaller warts may occasionally be confused with *Molluscum contagiosum.* Histopathologically, genital warts characteristically rise above the skin surface due to enlargement of the dermal papillae, have parakera-tosis and the characteristic nuclear changes typical of HPV infections (nuclear enlargement with perinuclear clearing). DNA based tests are available for diagnosis of HPV infections and for genotyping. Most of these are very resource intensive and expensive and hence not used in clinical care settings.

In recent times more options are becoming available for HPV testing to detect comment genotypes including those responsible for causing anogenital warts.

Treatment

Treatment for genital warts depends on the type of warts (nature of the lesion) and where they are located. The two main types of treatment for anogenital warts are:

i.   application of a cream, lotion or other appropriate chemical to the warts (topical treatment).
ii.   destruction of the tissue of the warts by freezing, heating or manual removal (physical ablation).

Most topical treatments tend to work better on softer warts, and physical ablation tends to work better on harder and rougher-feeling warts. Sometimes, a combi-nation of treatments is recommended. There are several topical treatments that can be used to treat genital warts.

- Podophyllotoxin is usually recommended to treat clusters of small warts. It comes in liquid form (0.5% solution) and works by having a toxic effect on the cells of the warts. A special application stick is used to draw up the liquid, which is then applied on to the wart. Treatment with Podophyllotoxin is based on cycles. The first treatment cycle involves applying the medication twice a day for three days. This is then followed by a rest cycle of about four days without treatment. Most people require four to five treatment cycles separated by rest cycles. The protocol in Ghana recommends application twice a day, three times in a week for a total of four weeks. Podophyllotoxin is contraindicated in pregnancy.

- 10-25% Podophyllin must be applied only to the wart as it will cause significant damage to normal skin. It is advisable to apply paraffin cream to normal surrounding skin before application of Podophyllin. There is need to wash the cream off within 1-4 hours after application. This treatment should be repeated at weekly interval.

- Imiquimod 5% is a type of cream usually recommended to treat larger warts. It stimulates the immune system to attack the warts. It is applied to the warts and then is washed off after 6 to 10 hours. This should be done three times a week for about 16 weeks.

- Trichloroacetic acid (TCA, 80-90%) may be recommended to treat small warts that are hard. It works by destroying the proteins inside the cells of the wart. But if it is not applied correctly, TCA can damage healthy skin. Hence it is essential to apply only to the wart and also protect surrounding healthy skin with protective gel before the application. TCA is thought to be safe to use during pregnancy.

There are four main methods used in the physical ablation of anogenital warts. These are:

- Cryotherapy: Involves freezing the wart using liquid nitrogen and is usually recommended to treat multiple small warts, particularly those that develop on the shaft of the penis, or near the vulva. Repeated applications are usually needed.

- Excision: Involves surgical removal of warts and is sometimes recommended to treat small hardened warts, particularly where this is a combination of smaller warts that have joined together. Excision can cause scarring, so it may not be suitable for large warts.

- Electrosurgery: Electrosurgery is a specialist treatment. It is often combined with excision to treat large warts that develop around the anus or vulva that have failed to respond to topical treatment. Excision is first used to remove the outer bulk of the wart. A metal loop is then pressed against the wart and an electric current is passed through the loop to burn away the remaining part of the wart.

- Laser surgery: Laser surgery is also a specialist treatment. It may be recommended to treat large genital warts that cannot be treated using other methods of physical ablation because they are difficult to access, for example, warts deep inside the anus or urethra. Laser beams are used to burn away the warts.

Prevention and Control

There are effective vaccines against HPV infection. These have been produced to offer protection against the most clinically relevant HPV types. Two of the vaccines available on the market include protection against HPV 6 and 11 and thus offer protection for anogenital warts. These are Gardasil (a quadrivalent vaccine) and Gardasil-9 (a nonavalent vaccine) can protect men and women from the most common HPV strains that cause genital warts, and also protect against strains of some hr-HPV to prevent cervical cancer. These are best given before girls and boys become sexually active and thus given around age 9-13 years in most developed countries. This vaccine is taken in 3 doses taken over 6 months.

In addition to the vaccine, safe sex practices are still essential to reducing risk. But it is worth noting although the use of condoms will generally offer protection against STIs, contact with other parts of the genital area unprotected by condoms can still lead to transmission of HPV, hence the use of condoms alone are not enough to offer protection against HPV/anogenital warts.

11

Human Immunodeficiency Virus

Aetiology

The Human Immunodeficiency Virus (HIV) is a retrovirus of the lentivirus genus and has an RNA genome. There are two main types, HIV-1 and HIV-2. HIV-1 has many sub-types and includes sub-types A, B, C, D, F and G. HIV infects CD4 positive T helper lymphocytes and replicates within the cells. The virus attaches to cells by using the gp120 envelope glycoprotein. The gp120 interacts with co-receptors including CCR5 and CXCR4. Following attachment, HIV enters the cell and goes through a cycle of viral replication. At the end of the cycle, new viruses are released which then infects new cells. The steps leading to viral replication described in Fig. 11.1 also indicates the key enzymes needed at each stage for replication. These enzymes have been the targets of antiretroviral drug designed to interfere with their activity.

Epidemiology

HIV/AIDS is a global problem. It is estimated that, over 35 million people are living with HIV worldwide, with two-thirds of them living in sub-Saharan Africa (SSA). Significant numbers of new infects are still being recorded especially in SSA. However, with the introduction of antiretroviral therapy and improved access to the drugs, AIDS-related deaths has significantly reduced. In Ghana, HIV infections shows a generalized epidemic

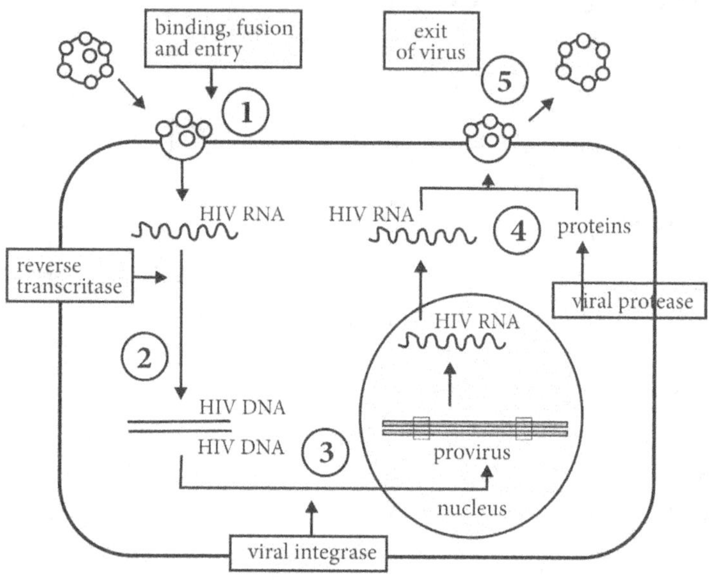

Figure 11.1: the HIV replication cycle. Credit: Medical Microbiology Simplified. 2nd Edition. Chapter 32: Retroviruses by Obiri-Yeboah D & Nuvor Victor. Page 216

pattern with an overall downward trend in prevalence across the 10 regions in the country.

The commonest mode of transmission of HIV is through sex (peno-vaginal, peno-anal, peno-oral and other forms). Since the virus is commonly found in semen and vaginal secretions. Other modes of transmission include mother to child transmission during pregnancy, labour, delivery periods and through breastfeeding as well as through exposure to blood, blood products and body fluids of persons infected with the virus, most impor- tantly through contaminated sharps and needles.

This virus disproportionately affects women than men. This may be due to various reasons including anatomical, biological and social factors. Biologically the semen is a more efficient means of transmitting HIV. Hence, transmission from an infected man to a woman is more efficient. Social factors include the fact that most women in the worst affected regions of SSA are less educated, may be unemployed, poor, lack bargaining power and may be vulnerable to sexual exploitation. Cultural norms like polygamy may also make women more at risk. The type of sexual act also affects the risk of transmission with anal sex having a threefold higher risk compared with vaginal sex. This is mainly because the rectal mucosal is easily bruised during anal sex and hence increasing the transmission rate. This explains the significantly higher prevalence of HIV among men who have sex with men (MSM).

The second most important means of transmission of HIV aside sex is mother to child transmission (MTCT). This can occur during the pregnancy, during the delivery process or through breastfeeding. Without any intervention, it is estimated that the risk of MTCT is up to 35-40%. In addition to sex and MTCT, HIV transmission occurs through infected blood and blood products. These may occur through sharing of needles among injection drug users, transfusion of infected blood and blood products. Occupational exposures among health workers may occur through injuries with infected sharps etc. but the risk of transmission is generally low and varies based on factors like the type of injury, the type of exposure (percutaneous or mucosal), and whether post exposure prophylaxis (PEP) protocol was followed or not.

Other factors, which increases the risk of HIV transmission and acquisition, include the presence of other sexually transmitted infections, particularly those causing genital ulcers such as chanchroid, syphilis, genital herpes and chlamydia. The WHO estimates that the presence of ulcerative sexually transmitted diseases increases the risk of HIV transmission by 10%-50% in women and 50%-300% in men. In general, however, all sexually transmitted infections including gonorrhea and hepatitis B increase the risk of transmission and acquisition of HIV.

Clinical Presentation

Acute HIV infection is associated with nonspecific symptoms like fever, fatigue, rash, headache, nausea, night sweat and flu-like symptoms. The duration between primary infection with HIV and progression to clinical disease manifestation and AIDS is on average 7.5 years with a range of 2-15 years. From the stage of AIDS, death is said to occur usually within 2 years without intervention. Figure 11.2 shows the relationship between the CD4 count and the viral load across the spectrum of HIV infection and AIDS. This relationship is inverse generally with a higher viral load leading to a lowering of CD4 count as is the case at the AIDS stage of the infection. Eventually, the patients develop symptoms of opportunistic infections when the CD4 count is low. Factors, which affect the rate of progression from infection to AIDS, include:

- Viral virulence (HIV-1 being more virulent than HIV-2).
- Age of the person infected (children progress faster).
- Nutritional status of the infected person (inadequate nutrition leads to faster disease progression).
- Co-infection with other viruses (e.g. Hepatitis B virus).
- Comorbidities (e.g. uncontrolled diabetes mellitus).

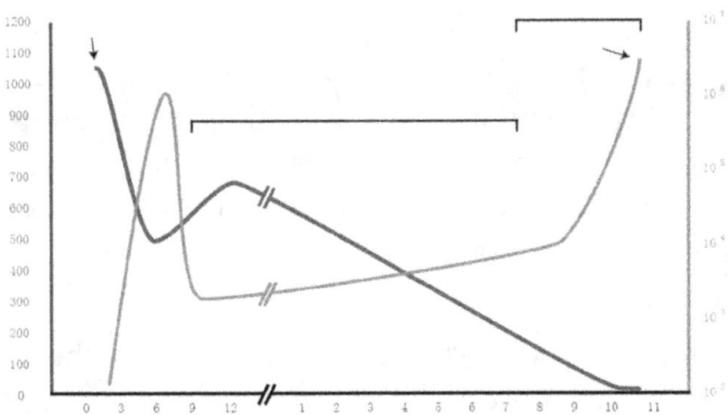

Figure 11.2: the inverse relationship between CD4 count and viral load. Credit: Medical Microbiology Simplified. 2nd Edition. Chapter 32: Retroviruses by Obiri-Yeboah D & Nuvor Victor. Page 216

In the primary infection stage, the CD4 count is high leading to a sharp drop in viral load in the early weeks of infection. By the clinical latency stage, there is some balance between the viral load and CD4 count, but over time, the viral load increases and CD4 count drops leading to signs and symptoms of AIDS. The World

Health Organization (WHO) classifies the progression of HIV infection to AIDS in four (4) stages. Tables 11.1 and 11.2 indicates the WHO staging system for adults and children respectively.

Laboratory diagnosis

Diagnosis of HIV infection is through either antibodies tests or detection of the virus itself. Currently, HIV diagnosis is mainly with rapid test kits. These detect antibodies to HIV-1, HIV-2 or both HIV 1/2 in whole blood, serum or plasma samples. The current HIV testing guidelines require three consecutive reactive tests from three different serological test kits, used sequentially, as the basis for HIV-positive diagnosis. If the first test is reactive but at most one of the subsequent tests is non-reactive, the result is described as indeterminate and should be repeated in 14 days. If it remains indeterminate, a tie-breaker nucleic acid test needs to be performed.

Although antibody testing offers rapid results, there are limitations to it's use and usefulness. The first limitation has to do with inability of the test kits to detect HIV infection during the window period; this being the period between when a person get infected and when enough antibodies have been produced to levels detectable by the test kits. The window period may range from 6 weeks to 3 months, and during this period, an infected person will not have developed enough an- tibodies to be detected by these rapid test-kits and thus resulting false negative results. The second limitation has to do with the uncertainty surrounding the outcome of HIV antibody testing in children less than 18 months.

Stages	Some associated clinical conditions
Clinical Stage 1	• Asymptomatic • Persistent generalized lymphadenopathy
Clinical Stage 2	• Pruritic Papular Eruptions • Herpes zoster • Recurrent oral ulcerations • Moderate unexplained weight loss (<10% of body weight) • Recurrent respiratory tract infections (otitis media, Sinusitis, pharyngitis bronchitis)
Clinical Stage 3	• Pulmonary tuberculosis • Persistent oral candidiasis • Unexplained chronic diarrhoea for longer than one month • Unexplained severe weight loss (>10% of body weight) • Oral hairy leukoplakia • Severe bacterial infections (e.g. meningitis, pneumonia, bone or joint infection, empyema, pyomyositis, severe pelvic inflammatory disease)
Clinical Stage 4	• *Pneumocystis jiroveci pneumonia (PCP)* • Extra-pulmonary tuberculosis • Recurrent severe bacterial pneumonia • HIV wasting syndrome • Cerebral toxoplasmosis • Cryptococcal meningitis • Oesophageal candidiasis • Kaposi sarcoma • Cytomegalovirus infection (retinitis or infection of other organs) • Progressive multifocal leukoencephalopathy • HIV encephalopathy • Invasive cervical carcinoma • Lymphoma (cerebral or B-cell non-Hodgkin) • Chronic cryptosporidiosis or Isosporiasis • HIV-associated cardiomyopathy or nephropathy

Table 11.1: WHO clinical staging of HIV/AIDS for adults (≥15yrs)

Stage	Some associated clinical conditions
Clinical Stage I	• Asymptomatic • Persistent Generalized Lymphadenopathy
Clinical Stage 2	• Herpes zoster • Recurrent oral ulceration • Unexplained persistent parotid enlargement • Extensive Molluscum contangiosum • Unexplained persistent hepato-splenomegaly • Recurrent or chronic upper respiratory tract infections (sinusitis, otitis media, tonsillitis) • Pruritic Papular Eruptions • Extensive wart virus infection
Clinical Stage 3	• Severe recurrent bacterial pneumonia • Pulmonary tuberculosis • Unexplained moderate malnutrition not adequately responding to standard therapy • Symptomatic lymphoid interstitial pneumonitis (LIP) • Unexplained persistent diarrhoea • Persistent oral candidiasis (after first 6 weeks of life) • Oral hairy leukoplakia
Clinical Stage 4	• *Pneumocystis jiroveci pneumonia* • Unexplained severe wasting, stunting or severe malnutrition not responding to standard therapy • Extra-pulmonary tuberculosis • Oesophageal candidiasis • Cerebral toxoplasmosis (after the neonatal period) • Kaposi sarcoma • HIV encephalopathy • Cryptococcocal meningitis • Cerebral or B-cell non-Hodgkin lymphoma • HIV-associated nephropathy or cardiomyopathy • Cytomegalovirus infection (retinitis or infection of other organs from >1 month old)

Table 11.2: WHO clinical staging of HIV/AIDS for children(<15 years with confirmed HIV infection)

Babies born to HIV-infected mothers are normally born with maternal antibodies acquire through the placental barrier during the period of gestation. These antibodies may persist up to 12-18 months in the newborn's blood may result in a false positive test outcome when the baby is tested prior to 18 months with an antibody test.

Viral RNA or DNA detection tests such as PCR assays are used to detect HIV infection in the window period (6 weeks - 3 months) when antibody tests will be negative. In Ghana, this test is also used for early infant diagnosis (EID) of babies born to infected mothers who are less than 18 months. Virological testing is also very essential in measuring response to antiretroviral therapy (ART) by indicating the viral load (copies/ml).

Treatment

Antiretroviral drugs (ARVs) have made a huge impact on the HIV situation globally by reducing AIDS associated mortality and morbidity, reducing MTCT of HIV etc. A combination of ARV drugs, usually a minimum of three drugs targeting different stages of the life cycle of the HIV are used in antiretroviral therapy (ART), to ensure effectiveness while also reducing the development of drug resistant strains. Commonly used ARVs (Table 11.3) in Ghana are selected from:

1. Reverse Transcriptase Inhibitors
    - Nucleoside Reverse Transcriptase Inhibitors (NRTIs)
    - Nucleotide Reverse Transcriptase Inhibitors (NtRTIs)
    - Non-Nucleoside Reverse Transcriptase Inhibitors (NNRTIs)

2.   Protease Inhibitors (PIs)
3.   Integrase Strand Transfer Inhibitors (INSTI)

Newer agents used in developed countries include entry and fusion inhibitors.

The international drive is towards treating all clients found to be infected with HIV irrespective of CD4 count, clinical stage or viral load. Individual countries have adopted the recommendations by WHO to suit their country specific setting to ensure sustainability of service delivery. Ghana has adopted WHO's 2015 guidelines that calls for initiating anti-retroviral therapy of all persons diagnosed with HIV irrespective of their WHO clinical stage or CD4 count provided they are willing and motivated to start treatment. The current ART guidelines of Ghana provides for this "treat all" approach. Where there are any limitations to implementing the "treat all" policy, ART must be prioritize to HIV positive clients based the following eligibility criteria:

a.   TB/HIV co-infected clients irrespective of CD4 count
b.   TB/HBV co-infected clients irrespective of CD4 count
c.   All Pregnant women irrespective of CD4 count
d.   All confirm infected children up to 18 years of age
e.   All infected clients in discordant relationships (the sexual partner is HIV negative)

4.   WHO clinical stage 3 or 4
5.   CD4 counts of ≤500/µl

ARV Class	Drugs	Dosage	Main side effect
NRTI	Zidovudine (AZT)	300mg 12hrly	Anaemia
	Abacavir (ABC)	300mg 12hrly	Hypersensitivity reaction
	Lamivudine (3TC)	150mg 12hrly	Generally safe
	Emtricitabine (FTC)	200mg daily	Generally safe
Nt RTI	Tenofovir (TDF)	300mg 24hrly	Renal impairment
NNRTIs	Efavirenz (EFV)	600mg daily	CNS effects from mild sleep disturbance to nightmares or psychosis
	Nevirapine (NVP)	200mg 12hrly	Skin rashes from mild to Steven Johnson Syndrome and also hepatotoxicity
PI	Lopinavir/ Ritonavir (LPV/r)	400/ 100mg 12hrly	Dysglycaemia
	Atazanavir/ Ritonavir (ATV/r)	300/ 100mg daily	Diarrhoea
INSTI	Dolutegravir (DTG)	50mg daily	Possible neural tube defect

Table 11.3: Commonly available ARVs in Ghana and their main side effects

Adherence counseling with a treatment monitor is encouraged before starting ART. These counseling sessions are repeated along the line as need may be to ensure continuous adherence and compliance. In Ghana, the preferred first line ARV drug regimen for ART is TDF + 3TC (or FTC) + DTG, since this regimen will cover most treatment scenarios, currently offers the best safety and efficacy profile, and reduces the pill burden due to availability of fixed dose combination formulation. All other possible regimen are considered alternative regimen, which can be used for specific patients to meet their needs. Second line regimen always include a PI in Ghana.

Factors which influence the choice of regimen include HIV type,consideration of potential side effects (see table 11.3), and other co-infections(TB-HIV and HBV-HIV co-infected patients requires EFV based regimen). In addition to the ARVs, HIV positive clients may have to take other medications as prophylaxis against some opportunistic infections. Co-trimoxazole 960mg daily for adults is mainly used as prophylaxis. Where cryptococcal meningitis is diagnosis, fluconazole is offered for treatment; followed by several months of secondary prophylaxis with fluconazole.

It is essential that all clients be monitored regularly to ensure prompt diagnosis and management of ARV side effects and most importantly treatment failure. Monitoring side effects require clinical assessment at each clinic visit and laboratory investigations including particularly, full blood count, renal and liver function tests at recommended intervals. Treatment failure in the context of ART is defined as viral load of more than 1000 copies/ ml in a client who has been on appropriate ART regimen for more than 9 - 12 months. It is essential to establish that such clients have been on the correct regimen and have been compliant. Despite the starting viral load, it is expected that the viral load will be less than 1000copies/ ml after 6 months of therapy and viral suppression (undetectable viral load) after 12 months. Since virological failure precedes immunological and clinical failure, the viral load test is essential. In Ghana, the policy therefore is to perform the first viral load testing 6 months after initiating ART, then at 12 months on ART with subsequent viral load testing every 12 months. Whenever virological failure is confirmed, such clients are changed to second line ART regimen and third line regimen when clients fail the second line.

Prevention and Control

There is currently no vaccine available for prevention of HIV infection. Following from the discussions on modes of transmission of HIV earlier discussed in this chapter, it should be evident that preventive measures for HIV transmission and acquisition must include measures targeting these. The measures include promotion of safer sex practices (the A, B, Cs), measures aimed at prevention of mother to child transmission (PMTCT), screening of blood and blood products, avoiding high risk practices like injection drug use and unsafe tattooing and the use of the standard precautions by health workers in caring for all patients.

PMTCT measures are targeted at all stages motherhood, pre-pregnancy, pregnancy, labour and delivery, as well as the post-delivery period. In summary, these PMTCT measure are:

- Educational campaigns to increase awareness among women and men to reduce HIV risky behaviors. This will help to reduce HIV prevalence generally in the population.

- Increasing access and availability of HIV testing points so that many people in the population will know their HIV status. The strategy of Family-Based Index Testing (FBIT) requires that the family members (sexual partners, children, parents and siblings as applicable) of all index clients be offered the opportunity to know their HIV status. It has been shown that the yield from such an approach is higher than seen through routine HTC. Thus, this FBIT approach has been adopted in Ghana too.

- Prevention of unintended pregnancies among HIV positive women through family planning education and access to services.

- Routine offer of HIV screening for all pregnant women to identify all HIV positive pregnant women.

- Use of ARVs by HIV positive pregnant women through all phases (pregnancy, delivery, post-delivery) and ARVs for exposed babies (In Ghana, the current protocol involving giving both Zidovudine and Nevirapine syrup for 12 weeks).

- Treatment, care and support for the woman, her partner through partner notification and screening services, her family and other children (screening of all children <18 years). This is supported by the FBIT as discussed earlier.

- Specific policies on delivery (in Ghana, vaginal delivery is still considered the safest mode of delivery for all including pregnant women living with HIV; caesarian section is only to be undertaken mainly on obstetrics grounds but not just based on HIV positive status).

- Specific policies on infant feeding especially policies on breastfeeding. In Ghana, HIV infected mothers still breastfeed exclusively for 6 months then continue breastfeeding with complementary feeds up to 12 months.

Post exposure prophylaxis (PEP) is essential for work place exposures for health workers and survivors of sexual defilement and rape. To achieve the best outcome, ARVs must be started as soon as possible after exposure, within 2 hours and unlikely to be effective if started after 72 hours. All exposures are assessed and classified based on the level of risk associated with exposure into very low, low and high risk. Factors that inform the classification of risk include the type of exposure (splash onto intact or abraded skin, mucous membrane splash, needle stick injuries, rape or defilement etc.), the HIV status of the source client among others.

It is also important that the HCW or exposed client is tested to establish the HIV status so that positive clients will not take prophylaxis but are linked for comprehensive care. It also enables negative status to be documented at baseline for future reference. Other baseline investigations include full blood count, renal function and liver function tests.

Very low risk exposure does not require the use of ARVs. This also uses triple therapy which includes a protease inhibitor for all exposures which qualify for ARVs (low and high risk exposures), and is taken for 28 days. It is important that the exposure client takes all the ARVs and follow the counseling on safe sex during this period. Follow up HIV tests and other tests will be carried out and the final HIV status for this exposure to determine the outcome will done at 6 months.

The strategy of the use of Pre Exposure Prophylaxis (PrEP) is also recommended and this has been adopted to varies levels in different countries. The considerations include the use of PrEP for partners of infected clients, sex workers and other high risk populations.

Hepatitis B Virus Infection

Introduction

Hepatitis B virus (HBV) is a double-stranded DNA virus of the hepadnaviridae family that establishes chronic infections leading to liver diseases and hepatocellular carcinoma. This virus is one of the important causes of viral sexually transmitted infections and is said to be responsible for 60-80% of hepatocellular cancers.

Epidemiology

HBV is distributed worldwide and its mode of transmission is through contact with infected blood and other body fluids like semen and vaginal secretions. Sexual transmission is common among heterosexual couples. Vertical transmission from infected mothers to the baby is very important particularly in Africa. Globally, regions of the world are grouped into areas of low prevalence (<2%), intermediate prevalence (2-8%) and high prevalence (>8%). Ghana and most parts of Sub Saharan Africa (SSA) are in the high prevalence zone. Following infection, about 90% of adults are able to clear the infection whereas among neonates and children only about 10 % are able to clear the infection (Figure 12.1 &Figure 12.2 respectively). This implies that infants and children when infected have a higher risk of progression from an acute infection to a chronic infection with the associated clinical conditions and sequelae such as cirrhosis and cancer of liver later in life.

Other factors which may contribute to persistence and progression of HBV include the immune status of the individual (co-infection with HIV) and genetic factors. Chronic infection is said to have occurred when the HBsAg is detectable after 6 months of infection.

Clinical presentation

The incubation period ranges from 40 – 180 days. The virus replicates in the hepatocytes and the inflammation response contributes to the damage to the liver. The recognized symptoms of jaundice are usually preceded by gastrointestinal symptoms such as nausea, vomiting, anorexia, abdominal discomfort and mild fever. The clinical conditions are classified as acute or chronic. Asymptomatic infections also occur. Chronic carriers who are clinically asymptomatic continue to be infectious. Some infected individuals (about 1 %) may get fulminant hepatitis and may die from an acute infection (Figure 12.1& 12.2).

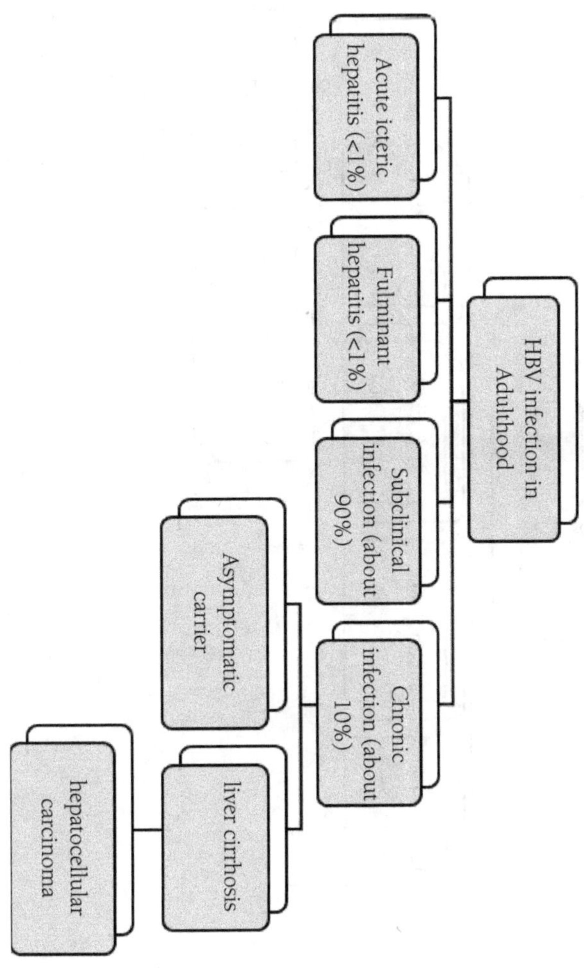

Figure 12.1: Natural history of HBV infection in people infected during adulthood

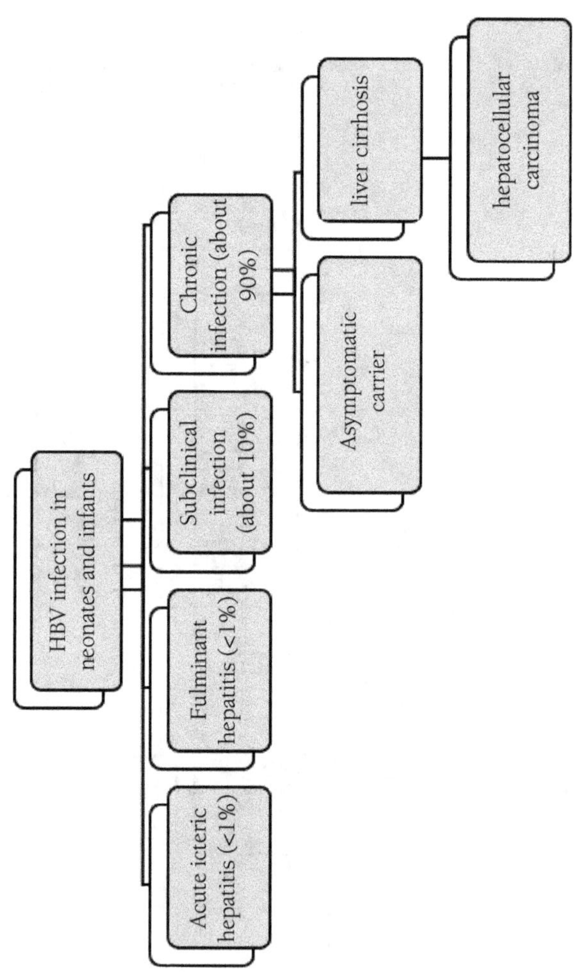

Figure 12.2: Natural history of HBV infection in people infected in utero, during perinatal and neonatal periods or in infancy

Laboratory diagnosis

Serology is the main method for diagnosis and Table 12.1 shows the immunological parameters and the possible interpretations of the results.

Molecular methods are commonly reserved for viral load estimation rather than routine diagnosis. Viral load estimation is essential in the decision to treat or not to start treatment in infected individuals and also help to indicate when therapy can be stopped. These polymerase chain reaction (PCR) based methods also offer opportunity to determine the specific genotypes an individual is infected with.

Liver function test, serum alpha fetoprotein, abdominal ultrasound and other laboratory investigations may be needed to determine the associated complications.

Treatment

Management of acute HBV hepatitis like most viral hepatitis is mostly supportive unless fulminant hepatitis requires aggressive and appropriate care to reduce the mortality associated with it.

Treatment of chronic HBV is not mandatory for all persons diagnosed as the decision to treat at any point in time is dependent on a combination of factors. These factors may include the age of the patient, presence of HBeAg, significantly raised liver enzymes particularly the alanine aminotransferase (ALT), presence of liver cirrhosis, HBV viral load and evidence and degree of liver inflammation as per liver biopsy or fibroscan (where available and indicated). Putting structure in the evaluation of patients and following existing guidelines

Immunological Parameter	Result	Possible interpretation
Hepatitis B Surface Antigen (HBsAg)	Negative	An individual was naturally infected and developed immunity
Hepatitis B Surface Antibody (Anti-HBs)	Positive	
Hepatitis core Antibody (Anti-HBc)	Positive	
Hepatitis B e Antigen (HBeAg)	Positive	Usually indicate active HBV replication and high infectivity.
Hepatitis B e Antibody- (HBeAb)	Negative	
HBe Ag	Negative	Usually indicate low HBV replication and low infectivity
HBeAb	Positive	
HBsAg	Negative	An individual was vaccinated and developed immunity
Anti-HBs	Positive	
Anti-HBc	Negative	
HBsAg	Positive	An acute infection of an individual
Anti-HBs	Negative	
IgM Anti-HBc	Positive	
IgG Anti-HBc	Negative	
HBsAg	Positive	A chronic infection of an individual.
Anti-HBs	Negative	
IgM Anti-HBc	Negative	
IgG Anti-HBc	Positive	

Table 12.1: Serologic diagnosis of viral hepatitis

would normally make decision taking and treatment easier. Upon proper evaluation and adherence to standard national/international guidelines most patients would be determined to fall into the category of patients who would not require treatment but just have to be followed up over a long period of time. Hence the decision to treat with drugs and the types of drug or drug-combinations to use must be taken carefully and done in accordance with existing guidelines.

Counseling of patients is essential to reduce anxiety and manage their expectations from any treatment or management decided upon. It should also be used to stress the importance of adherence and discuss potential side effects of treatment, possible treatment failure and avoidance of substances like herbal medications. For those who would not require treatment with antiviral agents, reassurance and need for regular follow up (6-12monthly) must be emphasized. It is essential to also discuss healthy lifestyle including adequate balanced diet and reduction or avoidance of alcohol.

It is important to start treatment at a time when it is needed without delay so as to prevent irreversible liver damage. Additional goals of treatment will be to possibly achieve virological clearance, improve liver function, HBeAg seroconversion and improve the overall quality of life of the patient. Thus, all patients with chronic HBV infection who have any one or more of the following conditions must be treated:

1. Patients with persisting abnormal ALT levels, HBV load >2000IU/ml and evidence of liver fibrosis (#APRI Score>2).

2. Patients with liver cirrhosis (decompensated or not) irrespective of ALT level.

3. Patients with viral load >20,000IU/ml and ALT >2 times the upper limit of normal.

#APRI is AST to Platelet Ratio Index and is used to predict whether there is significant liver fibrosis or cirrhosis. Online calculators are available to estimate the score.

Treatment can involve the use of immune system modulators like Interferon alpha (or Pegylated interferon which allows for weekly injections), antiviral agents such as Lamivudine (100mg daily), Emtricitabine (200mg daily) or Tenofovir dixopoxil fumarate. Currently use of single oral antiviral agents e.g. Tenofovir (300mg daily) is recommended for adults while Entecavir is preferred for children 2-11 years. Lamivudine has a higher rate of treatment failure and development of resistance hence not recommended as the first line treatment. Pegylated interferon alpha-2a (180μg once a week) is recommended for specific patients (excluding children <12 years) depending on factors including:

- severe inflammatory changes on liver biopsy
- very high ALT values
- moderately high viral loads
- some HBV genotypes

It is essential to monitor patients liver function and HBV load regularly (3 months after initiating treatment recommended). In addition those on Tenofovir will require renal function tests and for those of Pegylated interferon, HBsAg quantification. These labs would then be done at 12 weeks, 24weeks, 48 weeks and then annually as indicated.

Prevention and Control

The prevention of HBV involves several steps to avoid the transmission of the virus among individuals. These include safer sex practices, the use of the standard precautions by health workers in caring for all patients. It is essential that vaccination using the recombinant vaccine be used for everyone particularly in high endemic regions of the world such as sub-Saharan Africa. This requires that 3 doses be completed in the defined interval to ensure adequate protection. This vaccine is currently part of the immunization schedule for children in Ghana but there is a large pool of unvaccinated adults. It is essential that this large pool of adults are vaccinated to reduce vertical transmission as it ensures that mothers are protected.

To reduce risk of mother to child transmission, pregnant women should have viral load determined and be managed on antiviral agents (Tenofovir preferred) if indicated, then babies born to infected mothers are to receive the immunoglobulin injection (0.5ml or 200IU) within 72 hours of birth in addition to the birth dose HBV vaccine (within 24hrs). Breastfeeding is allowed. These babies are then put on the routine immunization and continue till completion of the childhood vaccination series and their HBV status confirmed at 9-18mths.

Bacterial Vaginosis

Aetiology

Bacterial vaginosis (BV) is considered not to be a typical sexually transmitted infection. It is a condition which arises due to disturbance in the normal flora of the vagina with depletion in the concentration of beneficial *Lactobacilli species.* Healthy vaginal microbiota consists of species which produce lactic acid keeping the pH between 3.5 - 4.5 in women between puberty and menopause. This acidic medium has antimicrobial property which inhibits the growth of pathogenic organisms. BV is associated with overgrowth of *Gardnerella vaginalis* which is said to create a biofilm that allows other opportunistic bacteria, particularly anaerobes to thrive. This results in local immune disruption and inflammation.*G. vaginalis* is a Gram variable coccobacilli.

Epidemiology

BV is the most common vaginal infection in women of reproductive age. BV is said to be most common in some parts of Africa and least common in Asia and Europe. Factors which have been recognized as contributing to the imbalance in the vaginal flora include the practice of douching, having multiple sexual partners, having female sexual partner, broad spectrum antibiotic use, and using an intrauterine contraceptive device among others. Consistent condom use and having circumcised male partners provide protection. It is possible for sexually inactive persons to develop bacterial vaginosis and the condition may also be seen in women after menopause. BV microbiotas have been found in male partners of infected females; on the penis, the coronal sulcus, and in the urethra.Uncircumcised male partners may act as a 'reservoir', thereby increasing the likelihood of transmitting the infection during sexual intercourse.

Clinical presentation

Common symptoms include abnormally increased vaginal discharge which is commonly described as having a "fishy smell". The discharge which is usually whitish or greyish in colour, coats the walls of the vagina and may be associated with a burning sensation. The condition is usually without significant irritation, pain, itchiness or erythema (redness); and asymptomatic infections may occur. Having BV increases the risk of infection by other sexually transmitted infections including HIV. It is also said to possibly increase the risk of preterm delivery among pregnant women. BV is also a risk factor for pelvic inflammatory disease.

Diagnosis

BV is often confused with a vaginal yeast infection or infection with *Trichomonas vaginalis.* To make a diagnosis of BV, a vaginal swab should be obtained and tested for:

- *A characteristic "fishy" odour on wet mount.* This test, called the 'whiff test', is performed by adding a small amount of potassium hydroxide to a microscopic slide containing the vaginal discharge. A characteristic fishy odour is considered a positive whiff test and is suggestive of bacterial vaginosis.

- *Loss of acidity.* To control bacterial growth, the vagina is normally slightly acidic with a pH of 3.8–4.2. A swab of the discharge is put onto litmus paper to check its acidity. A pH greater than 4.5 is considered alkaline and is suggestive of bacterial vaginosis.

- *The presence of 'clue cells' on wet mount.* Similar to the whiff test, the test for clue cells is performed by placing a drop of sodium chloride solution on a slide containing vaginal discharge. If present, clue cells can be visualized under a microscope. These are epithelial cells that are coated with bacteria.

These parameters are used in the Amsel's diagnostic criteria for BV. At least three of the four criteria should be present for a confirmed diagnosis. The components of the criteria are:

1. Thin, whitish or greyish homogeneous vaginal discharge.
2. Release of a fishy odour on adding 10% potassium hydroxide (KOH) solution.
3. pH of vaginal fluid >4.5.
4. Clue cells on microscopy.

Treatment, Prevention and Control

Usually treatment is with the antibiotics such as clindamycin or metronidazole which cover anaerobes. These medications may be considered safe for use in the second or third trimesters of pregnancy. The condition often recurs following treatment, and probiotics may help prevent re-occurrence. Recurrence rates are increased with sexual activity and inconsistent condom use. Hormonal contraceptive with and particularly oestrogen containing hormonal contraceptives, have been associated with a decreased prevalence of BV and decreased recurrence following management. A plausible explanation is the fact that such women were found to have improved vaginal flora and lactic acid level. Some steps suggested to lower the risk of BV include avoidance of douching and safer sexual practices.

Index

B

C

Cultural norms, **2, 57**
Cultures, **viii**
Cycle, **52, 55-56, 63**
Cytologic brush, **25**

D

Dacron, **25**
Daily infection, **viii**
Deafness, **4, 31**
Defilement, **2, 69**
Delivery, **8, 16, 24, 26, 28, 33, 45-46, 56-57, 64, 67-69, 81**
Developing countries, **1-2, 4, 15, 22, 29**
DFA, **26;** *see also Direct fluorescent test*
DGI, **18;** *see also Disseminated gonococcal infection; Gonococcal antimicrobial susceptibility programme*
Direct fluorescent test, **26;** *see also DFA*
Disclosure, **viii**
Discovery of syphilis, **viii**
Discrimination, **viii**
Disease, **16, 18, 22-23, 29, 32, 35, 39-40, 48, 58-59, 61, 81**
Disseminated gonococcal infection, **18;** *see also DGI; Gonococcal antimicrobial susceptibility programme*
DNA, **20, 37, 44, 47, 51, 63, 71**
Donovanosis, **3, 39-43**
Double-stranded DNA, **71**
Doxycycline, **27-28, 33, 43**
Drug, **10, 19-21, 37, 43, 47, 55, 57, 63, 66-67, 77**
Dysuria, **17, 23**

E

Ecto-parasites, **3**
Education, **11-12, 68**
Efficacy profile, **66**
Efficiency of transmission, **3**
Electrosurgery, **53**
ELISA, **26**
Endocervix, **25**
Erythromycin, **27-28, 37**
Examination, **6, 8, 18, 31, 36, 43**
Excision, **53**
Exploitation, **2, 57**
Exposure, **13, 15, 56-58, 69-70**
Eyelids, **17, 24**

K